PLANT BASED HEALING AND NUTRITION

FOR NOVICES

Discover The Healing Power Of Plants - A Holistic Approach To Wellness With Nutrient-Rich Foods And Transformative Lifestyle Practices

DR. TADEO KASEN

Table of Contents

DISCLIAMER

This book is intended for informational and educational purposes only. The content provided in this book is not a substitute for professional medical advice, diagnosis, or treatment. Always seek the advice of your physician or other qualified health provider with any questions you may have regarding a medical condition.

The techniques and practices described in this book are based on general principles and may not be suitable for everyone. Individual results may vary, and it is important to consult with a qualified healthcare professional before undertaking any new health or wellness program.

The author and publisher of this book are not responsible for any adverse effects or consequences resulting from the use of information, suggestions, exercises, or techniques presented herein. The reader assumes full responsibility for his or her actions and choices. The information provided in this book is accurate and reliable. However, the author and publisher make no representation or warranties of any kind, express or implied, regarding the completeness, accuracy, reliability, or suitability of the information provided.

Any References to specific products, services, or organizations do not imply endorsement or recommendation by the author.

By reading this book, the reader acknowledges and agrees to the terms of this disclaimer. If the reader does not agree with these terms, they should not use the information provided in this book.

CHAPTER ONE

Plant-Based Healing: An Overview

There has been a rising realization in recent years of the significant influence that plant-based healing and nutrition may have on our general well-being. This holistic approach to health stresses entire plant foods as a foundation for avoiding and treating a variety of health issues. The change to plant-based health is more than simply a dietary option; it signifies a way of life that embraces nature's healing ability.

The essence of plant-based medicine is the concept that by eating predominantly plant-derived foods, many chronic ailments may be alleviated or even reversed.

This break from traditional dietary rules is based on scientific data that plants are not only high in vital nutrients but also contain a plethora of bioactive chemicals with therapeutic capabilities.

The Vitality Of Whole Plant Foods

The potency of entire plant foods lies at the heart of plant-based healing. Whole plant meals, as opposed to processed foods, which frequently lack important nutrients and are heavy in harmful additives, contain a variety of vitamins, minerals, fiber, and antioxidants. This therapeutic paradigm is built on fruits, vegetables, whole grains, nuts, and seeds.

Whole plant meals are not only nutrient-dense, but they also provide several health advantages. The fiber in these meals enhances digestive health and aids with blood sugar regulation. Antioxidants, which are plentiful in colored fruits and vegetables, fight oxidative stress and inflammation, lowering the risk of chronic illnesses including heart disease and cancer.

Plant Foods High In Nutrients

Focusing on nutrient-rich plant meals to address the body's nutritional demands is one of the core concepts of plant-based therapy. Vitamins and minerals are abundant in leafy greens like kale and spinach, cruciferous veggies like broccoli and Brussels sprouts, and vibrant berries. Legumes, such as lentils and chickpeas, are high in protein, which is necessary for muscle upkeep and repair.

Plant-based eating is about plenty and diversity, not deprivation. Individuals may ensure a broad spectrum of nutrients by including a diversified selection of plant foods in their diet. This method not only promotes general health but also improves the immune system, making the body more resistant to sickness.

The Health Benefits Of Phytochemicals

Phytochemicals, which are naturally occurring molecules present in plants that contribute to their color, flavor, and disease resistance, are fundamental to the healing potential of plant-based diets. These bioactive substances, which include flavonoids, carotenoids, and glucosinolates, have several health advantages.

Flavonoids, which are found in berries, citrus fruits, and dark chocolate, for example, have antioxidant and anti-inflammatory qualities. Carotenoids, which are present in orange and yellow vegetables such as carrots and sweet potatoes, support eye health and immune system function. Glucosinolate-rich cruciferous vegetables have been associated with cancer prevention.

Understanding and using the potential of phytochemicals is a critical component of plant-based therapy. These chemicals not only contribute to the beautiful colors and tastes of plant meals, but they also play an important role in disease prevention and management.

Types And Variations Of Plant-Based Diets

Plant-based diets come in a variety of flavors to suit varied tastes and health objectives. The vegan diet, which avoids all animal products, is the most well-known. Vegetarian diets contain dairy and eggs, but pescatarian diets include fish. Flexitarian diets are adaptable, allowing for occasional meat eating.

Each type of plant-based diet has its own set of advantages. Vegans, for example, may have lower cholesterol and a decreased risk of heart disease. Vegetarians frequently benefit from better weight control and a lower risk of diabetes. Pescatarians benefit from omega-3 fatty acids found in fish, which promote brain and heart health.

Plant-based diets are accessible to a wide range of people due to their adaptability to individual tastes and cultural variances. Adopting a plant-based diet, whether prompted by ethical, environmental, or health concerns, is a customized journey that can be adapted to fit a variety of lifestyles.

Making The Switch To A Plant-Based Diet

Transitioning to a plant-based diet is a lengthy process that requires conscious and long-term changes. It is not about making drastic changes overnight, but rather about adopting a mentality that values progress over perfection. To guarantee a smooth transfer, follow these suggestions:

1. Educate Yourself: It is critical to understand the nutritional components of plant-based diets as well as the potential health advantages. This understanding provides people with the information they need to make smart food decisions.

2. Gradually increase the amount of fruits, vegetables, legumes, and whole grains in your diet. Your taste senses and digestive system can adjust to gradual alterations.

3. Experiment with Recipes: Take advantage of the wide range of plant-based recipes available. Experimenting with new flavors and culinary techniques makes the transition more joyful and aids in the discovery of new favorites.

4. Seek Help: Joining a community or seeking help from friends and family might help you stay

motivated. A friendly environment is created by sharing experiences, recipes, and advice.

5. Pay Attention to Your Body: Notice how your body reacts to the changes. Adjust your diet according to your energy levels, digestion, and general health.

6. Include Nutrient Supplements if Necessary: While a well-balanced plant-based diet can offer most nutrients, some components such as vitamin B12, vitamin D, and omega-3 fatty acids must be monitored. Supplements may be advised, particularly in areas with minimal sun exposure.

Finally, plant-based healing and nutrition reflect a paradigm shift toward a more holistic and long-term approach to health. This therapeutic concept is built on whole plant meals that are high in minerals and phytochemicals. Whether you choose a vegan, vegetarian, or flexitarian diet, the idea is to take it slowly and focus on information, experimentation, and individual choices.

Individuals may not only improve their physical health but also contribute to a more sustainable and compassionate society by utilizing the power of a plant-based diet.

CHAPTER TWO

The Effects Of Plant-Based Diet On Chronic Diseases

Plant-based nutrition has received a lot of attention in recent years, not just as a dietary option, but also as a powerful method for avoiding and controlling chronic illnesses. Chronic illnesses, such as heart disease, diabetes, and certain malignancies, have emerged as important public health issues across the world. Plant-based diets, which emphasize fruits, vegetables, whole grains, legumes, nuts, and seeds, have shown encouraging outcomes in lowering the risk factors for various illnesses.

One of the most important components of a plant-based diet is its beneficial effect on heart health. Plant-based diets have been shown in studies to lower blood pressure, cholesterol levels, and the risk of cardiovascular disease. Plant foods' high fiber content helps to preserve cardiovascular health by encouraging healthy blood vessels and lowering inflammation.

Furthermore, plant-based diets are frequently lower in saturated fats, which are established risk factors for heart disease.

Furthermore, a plant-based diet has shown promise in the management and prevention of diabetes. Complex carbohydrates present in whole plant diets break down more slowly, resulting in more stable blood sugar levels. This is especially important for people who have diabetes or are at risk of getting it. According to several research, eating a plant-based diet can enhance insulin sensitivity and reduce the incidence of type 2 diabetes.

Another area where a plant-based diet shows promise is cancer prevention. Fruits and vegetables include antioxidants, phytochemicals, and other bioactive components that have been associated with a lower risk of some malignancies. Cruciferous vegetables, such as broccoli and kale, contain chemicals that may aid in the inhibition of cancer cell proliferation.

Furthermore, the fiber in plant-based diets might help you maintain a healthy weight, which is an important component in cancer prevention.

In essence, a plant-based diet provides a comprehensive strategy for lowering the risk of chronic illnesses. It promotes general health and well-being by supplying a diverse variety of nutrients and antioxidants, functioning as a potent preventative tool against some of today's most pressing health challenges.

Specific Plants' Healing Properties

Nature has historically provided medicines, and individual plants have been recognized for their healing abilities throughout nations and traditions. For millennia, the medicinal potential of various plants has been recognized and employed, ranging from traditional herbal medicine to current scientific studies.

One noteworthy example is the aloe vera plant, which is well-known for its calming effects.

Topically applied aloe vera gel has been used to treat burns, wounds, and skin irritations. Because of its anti-inflammatory and antibacterial characteristics, it is an excellent natural therapy for encouraging skin healing.

Turmeric, a bright yellow spice produced from the Curcuma longa plant, is also a powerful healing herb. Turmeric's primary constituent, curcumin, has antioxidant and anti-inflammatory qualities. Curcumin may be effective in the treatment of illnesses such as arthritis, digestive issues, and possibly some forms of cancer, according to research.

The antibacterial effects of tea tree oil, which is extracted from the leaves of the Melaleuca alternifolia plant, are well documented. It has long been used to treat skin infections, wounds, and fungal infections. Because of the oil's antibacterial and antifungal properties, it has been used in a variety of cosmetics and pharmaceutical products.

Echinacea, a blooming plant native to North America, has long been used to stimulate the immune system. It is thought to boost the immune system and shorten the length and severity of colds and respiratory infections. Echinacea comes in a variety of forms, including teas, pills, and tinctures.

These examples demonstrate the many ways in which distinct plants aid in healing and well-being. These plants' unique components interact with the human body in ways that treat certain health conditions, providing a natural and often milder alternative to traditional pharmaceuticals.

Using Herbs And Spices For Health

Herbs and spices not only enhance the flavor of food, but they also have a major impact on health and well-being. Herbs and spices have long been used in culinary activities, with many civilizations acknowledging their therapeutic benefits. Incorporating a variety of herbs and spices into one's diet helps improve overall health.

Garlic, for example, is not only a tasty addition to recipes, but it also has various health advantages. It contains anti-inflammatory and antibacterial qualities, and it is thought to help cardiovascular health by lowering blood pressure and cholesterol levels. Garlic may also stimulate the immune system and deliver antioxidants, which help protect cells from injury.

Cinnamon is another spice that has amazing health benefits. It has been linked to better blood sugar management and insulin sensitivity, making it especially advantageous for people with diabetes or at risk of acquiring the illness. Cinnamon also has anti-inflammatory and antioxidant properties, which contribute to its ability to promote general health.

Herbs like basil, thyme, and rosemary provide more than simply flavor to dishes. These plants include anti-inflammatory and antibacterial essential oils and bioactive chemicals. They not only improve the flavor of foods, but they also give a natural approach to strengthen the body's immune system and reduce inflammation.

Turmeric, with its main ingredient curcumin, is a potent spice known for its anti-inflammatory and antioxidant properties. Integrating turmeric into various foods or taking it as a supplement can help with general health and may help with illnesses like arthritis and digestive ailments.

To summarize, herbs and spices are not just culinary embellishments, but also important components of a health-conscious diet. Their broad array of bioactive components can have a good impact on a variety of areas of well-being, making them a delightful and healthy addition to any meal.

CHAPTER THREE

Plant-Based Nutrition For Weight Loss

Obesity and weight-related health concerns have reached alarming proportions throughout the world, sparking an increased interest in effective and long-term weight control strategies. A plant-based diet has emerged as a potential approach to obtaining and maintaining a healthy weight.

The emphasis on full, nutrient-dense meals is one of the primary elements contributing to the efficacy of plant-based diets in weight management. Fiber-rich foods include fruits, vegetables, whole grains, legumes, nuts, and seeds, which increase fullness and help regulate hunger.

Plant-based meals, as opposed to processed foods, which are typically heavy in empty calories, supply important nutrients without adding extra calories, promoting weight reduction and maintenance.

The high fiber content of plant-based diets also plays an important role in blood sugar regulation. Stable blood sugar levels help to maintain energy levels and minimize cravings for sugary and processed meals, which aids in weight loss attempts. Furthermore, complex carbohydrates contained in plant meals break down more slowly, resulting in a more steady release of energy and a more sustained metabolic response.

Plant-based diets tend to be lower in harmful fats, especially saturated and trans fats. They instead give healthy fats like those found in avocados, almonds, and olive oil. These fats have been linked to a variety of health advantages, including better cardiovascular health and weight control. Individuals can minimize their calorie consumption while improving their overall health by selecting plant-based fats over animal fats.

Furthermore, a plant-based diet promotes conscious eating behaviors. The emphasis on entire foods, as well as the variety of flavors and textures, leads to a more fulfilling dining experience. This mindfulness can lead to a greater awareness of hunger and fullness cues, limiting overeating and assisting with weight loss objectives.

According to research, people who eat a plant-based diet have lower BMIs and are less likely to develop obesity-related disorders including type 2 diabetes and cardiovascular disease. A plant-based diet is a feasible and successful alternative for people seeking a healthy and balanced approach to weight management due to its long-term sustainability.

Plant-Based Diet For Mental Health

The relationship between diet and mental health is a growing topic of study, and evidence shows that plant-based nutrition can improve mental health. The complicated interplay between food intake, gastrointestinal health, and brain function emphasizes the necessity of a plant-rich, well-balanced diet for mental health.

Omega-3 fatty acids, which are found predominantly in fatty fish, flaxseeds, chia seeds, and walnuts, are essential for brain function. Plant-based diets can deliver these important fatty acids from plant sources, which can help with cognitive function and emotional well-being. According to research, omega-3 fatty acids may have antidepressant and mood-stabilizing properties, potentially lowering the risk of mental health issues.

Another way that plant-based eating promotes mental health is through the gut-brain link. The gut microbiome, a diverse population of bacteria in the digestive system, is involved in a variety of physiological processes, including those associated with mental health. Plant-based diets, which are high in fiber and varied plant chemicals, promote a healthy gut flora, which may improve mood and cognitive performance.

Fruits and vegetables high in antioxidants, which are cornerstones of plant-based diets, help the body fight oxidative stress.

Inflammation is connected to oxidative stress, and chronic inflammation is linked to an increased risk of mental health issues. Individuals may minimize inflammatory processes that may negatively influence mental well-being by lowering oxidative stress with a plant-based diet.

Furthermore, plant-based proteins such as beans, lentils, and tofu supply amino acids that are required for the production of neurotransmitters such as serotonin and dopamine. These neurotransmitters play critical roles in mood regulation, and appropriate production is critical for mental wellness.

To summarize, eating a plant-based diet has the potential to improve mental health through a variety of processes, including the provision of vital nutrients, support for healthy gut flora, and the decrease of oxidative stress and inflammation. Plant-based nutrition is emerging not just as a way of boosting physical health, but also as a comprehensive approach to supporting mental well-being, as research in this sector continues to advance.

Plant-Based Living's Ethical And Sustainable Aspects

Plant-based living is about more than just personal health; it is also about the health of the earth and ethical concerns. Adopting a plant-based diet is frequently driven by a desire to lessen one's environmental impact and encourage ethical animal welfare.

Environmental Longevity

The environmental effect of animal husbandry is one of the key reasons people switch to plant-based diets. Livestock farming substantially contributes to deforestation, water pollution, and greenhouse gas emissions. A plant-based diet rich in fruits, vegetables, grains, and legumes has a reduced carbon footprint and uses less land and water. Individuals may assist in saving natural resources and battling climate change by eating plant-based cuisine.

Animal Ethical Treatment

Many individuals are turning to plant-based diets owing to ethical concerns about animal cruelty in the food sector. Factory farming is frequently associated with overcrowded and filthy conditions, the systematic use of antibiotics, and brutal killing techniques. Individuals who live a plant-based diet match their decisions with compassion and respect for animal welfare. This transition benefits not just the animals but also the development of more humane and ecological agricultural techniques.

Eating Seasonally And Locally

Sustainable plant-based living extends beyond food selection to examine where and how those foods are produced. Choosing locally produced and seasonal vegetables helps local farmers while reducing the environmental effect of transportation. This option encourages biodiversity, benefits local economies, and builds a connection between people and their food sources.

Food Waste Has Been Reduced

Plant-based living is frequently associated with a greater awareness of food waste. When compared to animal products, fruits, vegetables, grains, and legumes have a longer shelf life. Individuals may minimize total food waste by adopting conscious consumption practices, so contributing to a more sustainable food system.

CHAPTER FOUR

Plant-Based Healing Meal Plans And Recipes

Plant-based healing is feeding the body nutrient-dense meals to promote overall health. Meal planning is essential for maintaining a balanced and enjoyable plant-based diet.

Nutrient-Dense Foods

A well-balanced plant-based diet has a wide range of nutrient-dense foods. Dark leafy greens, colorful veggies, whole grains, legumes, nuts, and seeds are all necessary. These foods are high in vitamins, minerals, antioxidants, and fiber, which help to boost immune function, energy levels, and general health.

Macronutrients In Balance

Plant-based meals should be carefully prepared to provide a macronutrient balance of carbs, proteins, and lipids. While plants contain proteins, combining them with other protein sources like beans and rice offers a full amino acid profile. Healthy fats like avocados, almonds, and olive oil assist to sustain satiety and support important biological activities.

Plant-Based Meal Varieties

A diversified selection of plant foods not only guarantees a wide range of nutrients but also improves the gastronomic experience. Experimenting with various fruits, vegetables, grains, and spices offers novel flavors and sensations, making plant-based eating more pleasurable and sustainable over time.

Eating With Awareness

Mindful eating is an essential component of plant-based therapy. Paying attention to hunger and fullness cues, savoring each meal, and eating in a comfortable setting will help with digestion and nutritional absorption. Furthermore, mindful eating promotes a healthy relationship with food, encouraging a holistic approach to health.

Recipes Made From Plants

There are several tasty plant-based dishes available that appeal to a wide range of tastes and preferences.

Individuals may explore a broad range of culinary choices, from nourishing salads to cozy stews and novel plant-based protein alternatives. Plant-based cooking websites, cookbooks, and cooking workshops give inspiration and direction for preparing healthful and delectable meals.

Surmounting Obstacles On A Plant-Based Diet

While plant-based living has many health benefits, it may be difficult to navigate social settings, manage nutritional problems, and locate convenient solutions. Overcoming these obstacles is critical for long-term plant-based diet adherence.

Considerations Of A Social And Cultural Nature

Gatherings and celebrations might provide difficulties for individuals following a plant-based diet. Open discussion about food choices with friends and family may foster understanding and support. Bringing plant-based foods to social gatherings guarantees that there are satisfying alternatives available and may even motivate others to experiment with plant-based eating.

Considerations For Nutrients

A plant-based diet requires proper consumption of specific nutrients, such as B12, iron, calcium, and omega-3 fatty acids. Supplements and fortified meals can help fill nutritional deficits. Individuals can adjust their plant-based diets to fit their unique nutritional needs by consulting with a healthcare provider or a licensed dietitian.

Accessibility And Convenience

Convenience is an important component in dietary choices in today's fast-paced environment. With a growing variety of plant-based items available in supermarkets and restaurants, plant-based eating is becoming more accessible.

However, preparing ahead, bulk cooking, and keeping simple snacks on hand might help people stick to their plant-based diet.

An abrupt move to a plant-based diet may be difficult for some people. Gradual transitions, such as implementing Meatless Mondays or gradually decreasing meat consumption, allow for changes in taste preferences and digestive capacity. This technique has the potential to make the transition more sustainable and pleasurable.

Plant-Based Nutrition For Every Stage Of Life

A plant-based diet is appropriate for people of all ages, including children, teens, adults, and the elderly. Maximum health must tailor the plant-based diet to fulfill the nutritional demands of each life stage.

Plant-Based Diets For Children And Adolescents

A well-planned plant-based diet can offer the nutrients required for growth and development in children and teens. It is critical to include a range of entire meals, including fortified plant-based alternatives for vital elements like calcium and vitamin B12. To enhance cognitive function and general health, parents should ensure enough protein, iron, and omega-3 fatty acid consumption.

Adult Plant-Based Nutrition

Plant-based eating can help individuals prevent chronic illnesses including heart disease, diabetes, and some malignancies. A diet rich in colorful fruits and vegetables, whole grains, and legumes promotes cardiovascular health, weight loss, and general well-being. Paying attention to specific dietary demands is critical for preserving vitality and longevity, especially as people age.

Plant-Based Diets For Seniors

Nutrient intake and metabolism may vary as people age. Getting enough minerals like vitamin B12, calcium, and vitamin D becomes even more important for bone health and overall well-being. A range of protein sources, such as beans, tofu, and plant-based protein supplements, can help seniors maintain muscular growth and strength.

Gut Health And Plant-Based Healing

The connection between plant-based nutrition and intestinal health is an important part of overall health. A plant-based diet high in fiber and plant chemicals supports a healthy gut microbiota.

Foods High In Fiber And Gut Health

Plant-based diets are naturally high in fiber, which is important for gut health. Fiber functions as prebiotic, feeding healthy intestinal microorganisms. Whole grains, fruits, vegetables, legumes, and nuts are high in fiber, which promotes regular bowel movements, prevents constipation, and promotes digestive health.

Plant Compounds And The Diversity Of The Gut Microbiome

The varied assortment of plant chemicals present in fruits, vegetables, and other plant-based diets helps to diversify the gut microbiota. A diversified microbiome is linked to better immune function, decreased inflammation, and a lower risk of developing numerous chronic illnesses.

A diverse plant-based diet encourages a thriving colony of healthy gut flora.

Anti-Inflammatory Effects

Many plant-based meals have anti-inflammatory qualities that help to maintain intestinal health. Chronic inflammation has been related to a variety of health problems, including digestive ailments. Polyphenols, which are present in berries, green tea, and dark chocolate, have anti-inflammatory properties, encouraging a balanced and healthy intestinal environment.

Foods High In Probiotics

Fermented plant-based meals deliver helpful probiotics into the diet. Sauerkraut, kimchi, miso, and plant-based yogurts include living cultures that promote digestive health.

Probiotics help to maintain healthy microbiota, aid with digestion and may improve nutrient absorption.

CHAPTER FIVE

Hydration And Digestive Function

Hydration is important for general health, including gut function. Drinking enough water aids digestion and helps avoid constipation. Herbal teas, infused water with fruits and herbs, and eating hydrating plant foods all help to maintain normal hydration levels in the stomach.

To summarize, adopting a plant-based lifestyle entails taking into account not just personal health but also the environmental and ethical ramifications of dietary choices. A comprehensive approach to well-being includes sustainable and ethical features, as well as attentive meal planning, recipe research, overcoming hurdles, and adjusting plant-based diets to different life phases.

Plant-based healing highlights the significance of a diversified and fiber-rich diet in sustaining a flourishing microbiome, particularly in the context of gut health. A careful and informed attitude may pave the way for a healthier, more sustainable, and happier existence as individuals negotiate the complexities of plant-based living.

Exercise's Role In Plant-Based Wellness

Plant-based wellness focuses on combining a plant-centric diet with a holistic lifestyle that includes frequent physical exercise. Exercise is essential for maximizing the advantages of plant-based nutrition and contributing to general well-being and health. This synergy between a plant-based diet and exercise is founded on preventative medicine and sustainable living concepts.

Metabolism and Physical Activity: Regular exercise supplements a plant-based diet by promoting healthy metabolic function. Because of the stronger thermic impact of digesting plant-based meals, plant-based diets rich in whole foods are known to enhance metabolism. This impact is increased when paired with exercise. Physical exercise boosts energy expenditure, assisting individuals in maintaining a healthy weight or, if necessary, losing weight. Furthermore, a plant-based diet combined with exercise has been related to enhanced insulin sensitivity, lowering the incidence of type 2 diabetes.

Cardiovascular health is an important element of general well-being, and plant-based diets and exercise both contribute considerably to heart health. Plant-based diets that are low in saturated fats and cholesterol have been linked to lower blood pressure and a lower risk of heart disease. Exercise enhances these advantages by increasing circulation, heart function, and vascular health. The combination of plant-based eating and regular exercise offers a robust barrier against cardiovascular disease.

Protein is needed for muscle growth and repair, and plant-based diets contain enough of protein from sources such as legumes, nuts, seeds, and tofu. Strength training workouts help to grow muscles even more. The amino acids included in plant-based proteins aid in muscle rehabilitation by lowering inflammation and boosting general musculoskeletal health. A balanced approach to fitness is fostered by the mix of plant-based nutrition and targeted activity.

Mental Health and Cognitive Function: Physical activity is helpful not just to the body but also to the mind. Endorphins, neurotransmitters that work as natural mood elevators, are released during exercise. When combined with a plant-based diet high in antioxidants and minerals, this combination has been shown to improve mental health. Plant-based diets may protect against sadness and anxiety, according to research. Regular exercise improves cognitive function, which leads to better attention, memory, and general mental clarity.

Considerations for the Environment: The link between plant-based well-being and exercise extends beyond human health to environmental sustainability. Plant-based diets have a lower ecological footprint than animal-based diets, which helps to conserve natural resources. Outdoor activities, such as hiking or cycling, allow people to connect with nature while also raising environmental awareness. The combination of a plant-based diet and eco-friendly workout options is consistent with a larger commitment to sustainable living.

In conclusion, exercise has a multifaceted function in plant-based well-being, spanning metabolic health, cardiovascular well-being, muscular growth, mental health, and environmental sustainability. A plant-based diet combined with frequent physical activity provides a healthy balance that supports general health and longevity.

Traditional Medicine And Plant-Based Nutrition

Plant-based nutrition is deeply rooted in traditional medical systems across the world, drawing on centuries-old traditions that acknowledge the healing benefits of plant-derived foods. Ayurveda, Traditional Chinese Medicine (TCM), and indigenous healing techniques all emphasize the interdependence of nature, the body, and total well-being. The incorporation of plant-based nutrition into traditional medicine represents a holistic approach to health that addresses not only illness treatment but also disease prevention.

Ayurveda: Ayurveda, an ancient Indian system of medicine, emphasizes the use of plant-based diets for balancing doshas (biological energies) and fostering optimal health. Plant-based nutrients play an important part in establishing this balance in the Ayurvedic diet, which is adapted to individual constitutions. With the notion that food is medicine, herbs, spices, fruits, and vegetables are recommended to address specific health conditions.

Traditional Chinese Medicine (TCM): TCM, which has been practiced for hundreds of years, incorporates plant-based nutrition as an essential component of health maintenance and illness prevention. Dietary suggestions frequently contain a range of plant-based foods such as herbs, mushrooms, and vegetables, reflecting the notion of balancing Yin and Yang energy. TCM acknowledges plants' therapeutic capabilities as well as their potential to balance the body's energy flow.

Indigenous Healing Techniques: Indigenous communities all over the world have their natural healing techniques. For feeding and healing, these techniques frequently incorporate the utilization of locally accessible plant-based foods. From Native American herbalism to African traditional medicine, there is a wealth of information passed down through centuries regarding the therapeutic virtues of plants. Plant-based nutrition is not just a source of nourishment in these situations, but also a source of healing and spiritual connection.

Phytotherapy and Herbalism: Herbalism, the use of plants for therapeutic reasons, is a common thread in traditional medicine throughout civilizations. Many contemporary medications are derived from plant components. Herbalism's holistic approach takes into account the synergistic effects of many plant chemicals, stressing the relevance of entire plant extracts rather than isolated components. Phytotherapy, often known as plant-based therapy, is the use of plant extracts to prevent and cure a variety of health problems.

Preventive Medicine: The emphasis on preventive medicine is one of the fundamental ideas shared by traditional medicine and plant-based nutrition. Both stress the importance of a well-balanced diet in sustaining health and preventing sickness. Plant-based diets, which are high in antioxidants, vitamins, and minerals, give the body the resources it needs to fight against ailments. Plant-based medicines are frequently prescribed by traditional medicine as preventative measures to preserve the body's homeostasis and increase lifespan.

In conclusion, including plant-based nutrition with traditional medicine shows a comprehensive and time-tested approach to health. Plant-based nutrition in traditional medicine emphasizes the intimate link between humans and the natural environment, advocating not just the treatment of diseases but also the promotion of total well-being.

Personal Plant-Based Healing Success Stories

The path to plant-based treatment is frequently highlighted by transformational personal experiences of people who have seen extraordinary changes in their health and well-being. These success stories are eloquent testimony to the potential benefits of adopting a plant-based diet. These stories, ranging from conquering chronic diseases to gaining robust energy levels, motivate people to investigate the therapeutic possibilities of a plant-based diet.

Weight Management and Metabolic Health: To address weight management and metabolic health concerns, many people turn to plant-based treatment. Personal success stories frequently include considerable weight loss, better blood sugar management, and increased metabolic performance. Plant-based diets that emphasize entire, nutrient-dense meals are a healthy and effective way to lose weight. Success stories usually emphasize the long-term character of these changes, which promote not only weight reduction but also general metabolic health.

Reversal of Chronic Diseases: Plant-based healing has been linked to the reversal of numerous chronic diseases. There are several stories of people who have effectively treated or even cured illnesses such as type 2 diabetes, cardiovascular disease, and autoimmune disorders by adopting a plant-based diet. Plant-based diets' anti-inflammatory qualities, together with their capacity to support healthy organ function, contribute to these favorable results. Personal anecdotes underscore the liberating change from symptom management to addressing the underlying causes of chronic illnesses.

Enhanced Energy and Vitality: The sensation of enhanced energy and vitality is a prevalent motif in personal success tales. Adopting a plant-based diet is frequently associated with reducing symptoms of sluggishness and weariness, increasing mental clarity, and improving general well-being. Plant meals high in nutrients give a consistent supply of energy without the energy crashes associated with processed foods. Success tales emphasize a renewed love for life and the capacity to engage in physical activities with zeal.

Improved Digestive Health: Digestive difficulties are a common worry for many people, and plant-based treatment may frequently provide relief. Success tales commonly explain how a plant-based diet helped people overcome illnesses including irritable bowel syndrome (IBS), acid reflux, and constipation. Plant foods' fiber content, along with their anti-inflammatory effects, promotes healthy gut flora and good digestive function.

Emotional Well-Being: A frequent issue in personal accounts is the relationship between plant-based healing and emotional well-being. People frequently relate experiences about how switching to a plant-based diet improved their mood, reduced anxiety, and increased brain clarity. The influence of a plant-based diet on neurotransmitters and hormonal balance is mentioned as a component of these good improvements. Success stories demonstrate the comprehensive nature of plant-based medicine, which addresses both physical and mental well-being.

Finally, personal success stories of plant-based healing demonstrate the transforming power of adopting a plant-centric lifestyle. These stories motivate and encourage others to investigate the significant influence of plant-based diets on numerous areas of health. These tales demonstrate the healing potential of plant-based living, whether the objective is weight loss, chronic illness reversal, greater energy, digestive health, or mental well-being.

Conclusion

To summarize, the acceptance of plant-based healing and nutrition reflects a paradigm change in our approach to health and well-being. A growing amount of scientific data suggests that a plant-based diet can help prevent and even reverse chronic illnesses including heart disease, diabetes, and some forms of cancer. Aside from the physiological benefits, adopting plant-centric diets has been related to improved mental health, increased vigor, and long-term weight control.

Plant-based nutrition's holistic character, rich in a broad variety of vitamins, minerals, and antioxidants, promotes a synergistic interaction between the body and the food it consumes. This nutritional approach stresses whole, unprocessed foods, creating a balance that goes beyond simply nourishment to the development of a flourishing ecosystem within the body.

Furthermore, the environmental benefits of a plant-based diet cannot be emphasized. As we battle with the effects of climate change, plant-centric eating emerges as a responsible choice that decreases our environmental impact. Individuals who choose plant-based therapy and nutrition benefit not just their health but also the health of the world.

Plant-based therapy and nutrition, in essence, signal a paradigm change toward a more compassionate, sustainable, and health-conscious world. The enormous influence on human well-being and the global ecosystem is set to generate a healthier, more peaceful future as knowledge rises and individuals make educated choices.